After Myomectomy

Post- Myomectomy Guidelines and Dietary Requirements for Full Recovery made Handy.

By

CYNTHIA LEONARD

CHAPTER 1: Understanding Myomectomy

Uterine fibroids, also known as leiomyomas or myomas, are removed surgically in a surgery called a myomectomy. These non-cancerous growths appear on the uterus's muscular wall. Women with symptomatic fibroids who want to maintain their uterus or increase their fertility are often advised to undergo a myomectomy. *Here is a thorough explanation of myomectomy:*

Myomectomy is often advised when fibroids result in symptoms including excessive monthly flow, pelvic discomfort, pressure on the bladder or rectum, or problems with fertility. Women who desire to keep their uterus for potential childbirth or other personal reasons are given consideration.

Myomectomy Types:

Abdominal Myomectomy: The typical method of myomectomy involves making an incision in the abdominal wall to get access to the uterus. For bigger or more numerous fibroids, it is used.

Laparoscopic Myomectomy: This minimally invasive procedure uses a camera (laparoscope) to direct the surgeon while requiring less incisions. It gives faster healing times and is suited for smaller fibroids.

Hysteroscopic Myomectomy: Least intrusive technique, hysteroscopic myomectomy, is appropriate for fibroids that are mostly located within the uterine cavity. The fibroids are accessed and removed with a hysteroscope.

Preparation:

To ascertain the position, size and quantity of fibroids, you will normally undertake a variety of tests before myomectomy, including imaging exams like ultrasound or MRI. Additionally, your health and medical background will be evaluated.

Process:

Depending on the size, location and experience of the surgeon, a particular process and technique will be performed. The healthy uterine tissue is kept intact when the fibroids are removed throughout the procedure.

Recovery:

Abdominal myomectomy: There will be some scarring from the incision and recovery might take several weeks.

Laparoscopic myomectomy: Recovery is often quicker and scarring is less.

Hysteroscopic myomectomy: There are no exterior incisions, and recovery is often speedier.

Myomectomy has hazards, including infection, haemorrhage, damage to nearby tissues and the development of scar tissue, much like any surgical treatment. You should go through these risks with your physician.

Fertility: By eliminating fibroids that were impeding conception or causing repeated pregnancy losses, myomectomy may enhance fertility for certain women. The amount of fibroid removal and other fertility parameters, among other things, have a role in the effectiveness of fertility improvement.

Following a myomectomy, you will schedule routine follow-up visits with your doctor to check on your progress and determine if any fibroids may have returned.

Alternatives: If fertility preservation is not a priority, a hysterectomy *(removal of the whole uterus)* may be an option instead of a myomectomy, depending on your unique circumstances and choices. Uterine artery embolisation (UAE) is a procedure that blocks the uterine artery.

For the best course of action to your particular condition and requirements, you must speak with a gynaecologist for fibroid management experts. They will provide you with comprehensive details on the advantages and disadvantages of myomectomy so you can decide on your course of therapy with confidence.

CHAPTER 2: Importance of Post-Myomectomy Recovery

For those who have had myomectomy surgery to remove uterine fibroids, post-myomectomy recovery is a crucial stage in the therapeutic process. Several factors make this recuperation phase crucial:

Healing and tissue repair: Myomectomy, a surgical operation, includes the removal of uterine fibroids. Incisions are formed and tissue is worked on throughout the procedure. During the healing phase, the body has time to restore and rebuild these tissues. For the risk of problems to be as low as possible, proper healing is crucial.

Pain management: Postoperative discomfort and pain are frequent. Recovery enables people to control their pain using medications and other methods suggested by their healthcare professionals. An easier and more pleasant healing process depends on effective pain management.

Cutting Down On Infection Risk: Infection is a possibility during surgery. The risk of infection is decreased with the use of proper post-surgical care, such as wound care and cleanliness. During the healing process, it's crucial to follow the doctor's instructions for wound care and, if required, take recommended antibiotics.

Healthcare professionals keep an eye out for difficulties throughout the healing process, such as heavy bleeding, fever or unusual discharge. Early identification and timely medical care may stop issues from becoming worse.

Returning to Regular Activities: Patients must have time to relax before gradually returning to regular activities. People are urged to refrain from heavy lifting, intense exercise and other activities that might put pressure on the surgical site while they are recovering. This encourages healthy recovery.

Emotional Health: Going through recovery may be difficult emotionally. Various emotions, such as worry and despair, may be experienced by patients. For mental well-being throughout this time, assistance from loved ones and medical professionals is crucial.

Fertility considerations: Those hoping to become pregnant in the future, the healing phase is crucial to allowing the uterus to repair and resume normal function. For a safe and effective recovery plan, it is crucial to discuss reproductive objectives with the healthcare professional.

Follow-up Care: After myomectomy recuperation, you'll have follow-up visits with medical professionals. These visits are essential for keeping track of the patient's progress, correcting any issues, and confirming that the patient is recovering as anticipated.

Patient education: Following surgery, patients are given information on how to care for themselves, including directions on nutrition, medicine and any restrictions or limits. For a good recovery, it is essential to be educated and to follow these guidelines.

Long-Term Health: Although myomectomy treats uterine fibroids immediately, it's crucial for patients to preserve long-term health. To avoid the return of fibroids, conversations regarding lifestyle modifications, contraceptive methods, and future intentions for reproduction often take place throughout the healing process.

CHAPTER 3: Purpose of These Guidelines

Guidelines for post-myomectomy care are meant to provide patients and medical professionals an organised list of suggestions and instructions to follow in order to guarantee a good recovery and reduce any possible consequences. Myomectomy, a surgical operation to remove uterine fibroids *(noncancerous growths in the uterus),* may be carried out using open surgery, laparoscopy or hysteroscopy, among other techniques. These recommendations are particular to the kind of myomectomy done and the patient's unique situation.

Here are some of the main goals of post-myomectomy recommendations:

- The main objective of the following recommendations is to ensure that the surgical site *(or sites)* where the fibroids were removed recovers correctly. Infections

may be avoided, discomfort and agony are
reduced and scarring is kept to a minimum.

- Post-myomectomy guidelines include
  advice on how to keep an eye on and deal
  with any issues including infection, excessive
  bleeding or damage to adjacent structures
  during the operation.

- Instructions on how to manage pain,
  including how to take painkillers and
  techniques to lessen discomfort after
  surgery, are often included in guidelines.

- Restrictions on intense activities, carrying
  heavy things and driving are included in the
  recommendations about physical activity in
  order to avoid strain or damage during the
  healing period.

- Recommendations may be made on diet
  and nutrition to promote recovery and
  prevent constipation, which is a typical
  problem after surgery.

- Instructions often include a plan for further visits with the doctor or other healthcare professional to check on healing, have any stitches or staples removed and to talk about any issues or problems that could come up.

- Plans for future pregnancies and fertility preservation may be included in the recommendations, depending on the patient's age, reproductive objectives and the kind of myomectomy that was done.

- Recognising the emotional effect of surgery, these recommendations could also provide patients with information on counselling or support groups to assist them deal with the emotional elements of recovery.

- To help patients make educated choices regarding their reproductive health, advice on contraception and family planning may be offered following myomectomy.

- Some patients may have fibroid recurrence, recommendations may call for routine monitoring to catch any new growths early on.

Preoperative Consultation:

The first stage in every surgical procedure, including a myomectomy, is a preoperative consultation. Uterine fibroids are benign growths that form in the uterus and are surgically removed during a myomectomy. This consultation, which is often held by a gynaecologist or a surgeon, serves to verify that the patient is adequately prepared for the treatment and that all pertinent data has been acquired to assure its safety and success. You may anticipate the following at a preoperative consultation for a myomectomy:

Examining the medical past:

The physician will begin by going over your medical background, including any ongoing illnesses, prior operations, drugs you are presently taking, and any allergies you may have. To protect your safety during operation, be truthful and as specific as you can.

Examining the Body:

You will get a physical examination to determine your overall health. To determine the size and location of your fibroids, a pelvic examination, blood pressure monitoring and heart rate monitoring may be used.

Surgical Procedure Discussion:

The myomectomy process will be thoroughly explained by the surgeon, along with the kind of myomectomy that will be done *(laparoscopic, abdominal or hysteroscopic)* and the anticipated results. They will also go through any possible hazards and problems that can arise during the procedure.

Anaesthesia:

You'll talk about whether general anaesthesia or local anaesthesia combined with sedation will be utilised for the surgery's anaesthesia. Your medical history may also be examined by the anesthesiologist to guarantee that anaesthesia will be provided safely.

Acknowledged Consent:

An informed consent form that you must sign demonstrates that you are aware of the advantages and disadvantages of the procedure as well as any available alternative therapies. Your acceptance of the myomectomy procedure is shown by this document.

Instructions for the Procedure:

The surgeon will give you specific preoperative instructions, such as advice on fasting before surgery, drugs to avoid and any required preoperative preparations *(such as bowel preparation for abdominal myomectomy)*, in addition to any essential preoperative medications. Imaging and lab tests

To offer more information for the procedure, you could be required to undertake diagnostic tests like blood work, imaging studies like an **MRI**, or imaging studies like an ultrasound.

Questions and Issues:

This is your chance to voice any queries or worries you may have about the operation, the healing process, or postoperative care.

Making Plans for Recovery:

The surgeon will go through the healing process in detail, including postoperative pain control, activity limitations and follow-up consultations.

Support System:

It's typical to feel anxious or stressed before surgery. The medical staff will provide emotional support and respond to any inquiries to assist allay your worries.

Home Preparation:

To guarantee a safe and effective operation and recuperation, there are some crucial procedures to take before having a myomectomy, a surgical treatment to remove uterine fibroids. Before your myomectomy, you may want to consider the following at home:

Your Healthcare Team should be consulted:

Make a preoperative meeting with your surgeon to go through the surgery, any worries or questions, and to get personalised instructions.

Any prescription drugs you must take before the procedure should be taken exactly as prescribed by your doctor. It could also include drugs to treat inflammation, control pain or stop infections.

Lifestyle Changes:

In the weeks before surgery, refrain from drinking alcohol and giving up smoking since these activities might hinder recovery.
To improve your general health, follow a healthy diet and exercise regimen. Your body's capacity for healing may be enhanced as a result.

Home Preparation:

Set up your living area such that it is cosy for your rehabilitation. To minimise leaning over, keep objects that are commonly used at waist or chest height.

Create a space in your home, such as your bedroom, where you may relax and heal. Think about stocking a nightstand or table with necessities like water, prescription drugs, and entertainment.

System of Support:

Make plans for a friend or family member to remain with you for a short time after surgery to help with domestic duties and provide emotional support. Give someone close to you the day and place of your procedure so they can help if anything happens.

Transportation:

Make sure you have a safe way to get to and from the hospital the day of the procedure. Following the treatment, you'll probably be unable to drive yourself home.

Diet before Surgery:

Any dietary guidelines given by your surgeon or anesthesiologist should be followed. Usually, you will be instructed to abstain from food and liquids before surgery.

Individual Hygiene:

According to your surgeon's instructions, take a shower or bath the evening before or the morning of your operation. On the day of the procedure, avoid using lotions, fragrances or cosmetics.

Dress Comfortably and Loosely:

On the day of your operation, wear comfortable, loose-fitting attire to the hospital. Something simple to put on and take off is what you need.

Mentally Preparing:

Utilise breathing exercises, deep breathing methods, or meditation to manage anxiety and stress. The rehabilitation process might be aided by an optimistic outlook.

Effective Communication:

Make sure you comprehend all pre-operative instructions, and have the contact information for your surgeon or the medical staff handy in case you have any questions or concerns before the procedure.

Preoperative Exams:

Perform any pre-operative screenings or testing that your surgeon requests, such as imaging or blood tests.

Monetary and Insurance:

Examine your financial plans and insurance coverage to make sure you are ready to meet any medical costs.

Effective communication with your medical team is crucial for a successful procedure and recovery, as individual needs may vary based on your health and the type of myomectomy.

Pre- Myomectomy Support System:

The pre-myomectomy support network is described as follows:

Your medical team is your support system's first and most crucial component. The gynaecologist, surgeon and anesthesiologist are all included in this. The process, its dangers, advantages and alternatives will all be explained to you by them. Additionally, preoperative evaluations will be done to make sure you are healthy enough for the procedure.

It's also crucial to educate oneself about the surgery, its consequences and the healing process. In addition to giving you educational materials and addressing any questions or worries you may have, your medical staff should be there to assist you.

Kin and Acquaintances: Utilise the emotional support of your loved ones. Discuss your worries and apprehensions with them and let them know how they can support you while you heal.

Support Groups: Getting involved in a support group for women who have had myomectomy surgery or are getting ready for it may be very beneficial. These groups may be found online or in person and they provide a venue for exchanging stories, getting answers to questions and receiving emotional support from others who have gone through similar circumstances.

Mental Health Support: If you're feeling worried or stressed out about the surgery, consider getting help from a therapist or counsellor. They may provide coping mechanisms and emotional support to aid in your emotional management.

Nutrition and Exercise: Before the procedure, discuss your diet and exercise regimen with your healthcare physician. An easier recovery may result from maintaining a healthy lifestyle, which may enhance your general health.

Plan for both the **Financial and Logistical** sides of the procedure. Understanding your insurance's coverage, making travel arrangements to and from the hospital and making sure you have the tools you need for a speedy recovery at home are all included in this.

Advance Directives: Talk to your family about your medical preferences and wants, also think about completing advance directives, such a living will or a healthcare proxy, in case there are unanticipated problems after surgery.

Preoperative Consultations: Show up on time for all preoperative consultations. The completion of any required tests or assessments, as well as your readiness for the operation, depend on you keeping these appointments.

Self-Care: In the days before the procedure, engage in self-care. As much as you can, control your stress while getting enough rest and eating healthily. You'll be in the greatest physical and mental shape possible when you have the procedure thanks to this.

CHAPTER 4: Post-Operative Period - Recovery Room Stay and Pain Management.

The post-operative healing phase is essential for a good result. *What to anticipate from the recovery room stay and pain treatment is as follows:*

Rehab Room Stay:

After the myomectomy, you will be sent to the recovery area for monitoring. Your vital indicators, including heart rate, blood pressure and oxygen levels, will be monitored by medical personnel in the recovery room. This observation makes sure that you are stable and that your anaesthesia recovery is going well.

Following surgery, you could feel some discomfort and pain. To keep you comfortable, nurses will evaluate your degree of discomfort and provide you medicine as necessary.

Controlling nausea: Vomiting and nausea are occasionally brought on by anaesthesia. If needed, medication may be used to control this.

As soon as you are awake, attentive and stable, you will stay in the recovery room. Usually, this takes many hours. The medical team will evaluate your health and determine if you are fit to be transferred to a normal hospital room or sent home after release.

Following surgery, Pain Management:

Prescription drugs: To treat post-operative pain, your doctor may recommend opioid painkillers *(such as oxycodone).* Follow your doctor's instructions while using these drugs. It's crucial to take your medicine as directed and not wait until the pain is unbearable since it works better that way. Ibuprofen and paracetamol are examples of over-the-counter painkillers that your doctor could suggest in addition to prescription drugs. To assist control discomfort, they may be used as instructed.

Ice packs may aid with edema reduction and some pain relief when placed on the abdomen region. Use a towel or cloth between the ice pack and your skin to avoid frostbite.

Relaxation and Rest: During the healing process, rest is crucial. For the period of time prescribed by your surgeon, refrain from intense activities, lifting and sexual activity.

Nutrition and Hydration: Maintaining a healthy weight while eating a balanced diet will help the body repair. Avoid alcohol and coffee since they might dehydrate you and possibly cause prescription interactions.

Attend all planned follow-up visits with your healthcare practitioner to keep track of how your recuperation is coming along. If you suffer severe or escalating pain, excessive bleeding, fever or any other odd symptoms, call your physician right once.

Monitoring Vital Signs and Potential Complications

To protect the patient's safety and enable early identification of any possible issues, post-operative monitoring is essential after a myomectomy. *Here is a list of vital indicators to watch and possible problems to look out for:*

1. Vital Signs:

Blood Pressure: Check your blood pressure often to look for changes. Pain or the stress of surgery may both cause hypertension.

Heart Rate: Pay attention to the patient's heart rate. Tachycardia *(rapid heartbeat)* may be a sign of discomfort or other issues.
The patient's respiratory rate and pattern should be evaluated. Modifications may indicate respiratory discomfort or suffering.

Body Temperature: A fever may be an infection. Regularly check your body temperature.

Measure Oxygen Saturation using a pulse oximeter to make sure that the blood has enough oxygen.

2. Pain management:

- Gauge pain intensity using a pain scale. For patients' comfort and recuperation, adequate pain management is crucial.
- Administer painkillers as directed by the doctor or other healthcare professional.

3. Surgical Site Monitoring:

a. Examine the surgical incision site for infection-related symptoms such edema, warmth, redness or discharge.

b. Check for any indications of a hematoma or a wound dehiscence, which is the separation of the wound's margins.

c. Look for indications of excessive bleeding or the development of hematomas, such as increased drainage on dressings.

4. Urinary Output and Bowel movement: To
maintain appropriate kidney function, monitor
urine output, including movement of the bowel.

- Urinary retention is a potential problem; if
  the patient has trouble voiding,
  catheterization may be necessary.

- Assess bowel movements and keep an eye
  out for any symptoms of postoperative
  ileus, which is a temporary paralysis of the
  intestines.

- Promote as much oral intake and early
  walking as tolerated.

Respiratory Status: In order to avoid atelectasis
(lung collapse) and pneumonia, evaluate lung
sounds and urge deep breathing exercises.

b. Keep an eye out for respiratory distress
symptoms including shortness of breath or oxygen
saturation.

5. Thromboembolic Events: Patients who have had a myomectomy are at risk of blood clots. Encourage early walking, using compression socks, and taking prescribed prophylactic anticoagulants.

6. Preventing Infections:

a. Keep an eye out for symptoms of infection, such as fever, a worsening of the surgical site's discomfort, purulent discharge, or generalised symptoms.

b. Give recommended preventive antibiotics as directed.

7. Neurological Status: Assess neurological function, such as awareness and orientation, to find any neurological difficulties.

8. Hydration and Nutrition:

a. Make sure you're getting enough fluids, and keep an eye out for any indications of dehydration.

b. Start a clear liquid diet and progress as tolerated, as directed by your doctor.

II. Psychosocial Support: Assist the patient's emotional needs and educate them about the healing process and also respond to the patient's queries or concerns.

9. Planning for Discharge:

a. Plan for the patient's discharge as soon as possible after surgery.

b. Ensure the patient is taking the right painkillers, is adhering to the prescribed course of action and is aware of any activity limits.

Issues that Might Arise:

- Infection Haemorrhage
- Anaesthesia-related side effects
- DVT *(deep vein thrombosis)* and PE *(pulmonary embolism)*
- Wound healing slowly
- Intestinal blockage or ileus
- Retention of urine
- Developing a seroma or hematoma
- Development of scar tissue
- Alterations to the menstrual cycle or fertility *(long-term issues)*.

CHAPTER 5: First Days at Home - Discharge Instructions

Medications and Pain Management

Here are a few typical directives:

Medications:

Prescription Painkillers: Your doctor may recommend painkillers to treat your post-operative pain. As prescribed by your surgeon, take these drugs.

Over-the-Counter Painkillers: In certain circumstances, your doctor may suggest using acetaminophen *(Tylenol)* or ibuprofen *(Advil)* over-the-counter to treat minor discomfort. Be careful to adhere to the suggested dose listed on the label or as instructed by your healthcare practitioner.

Antibiotics: Follow the instructions on any antibiotics your surgeon recommends to avoid contracting an infection.

Stool Softeners: Since painkillers might make you constipated, your doctor could advise stool softeners to help you avoid this problem. Observe the dose indicated.

Anti-nausea Drugs: Your doctor may recommend anti-nausea drugs if you have nausea or vomiting.

Iron Supplements: If you were anaemic before surgery or had blood loss during the treatment, iron supplements may be recommended to aid in your recovery.

Birth Control: If your doctor recommended birth control prior to surgery to treat your disease, talk to them about when and how to start using it again.

Follow-Up Appointments: Be careful to show up to any planned follow-up consultations with your surgeon to track your healing and resolve any issues.

Managing Pain

Rest: You should place a priority on rest in the first days after a myomectomy. Get plenty of rest, and steer clear of rigorous activity.

Ice: For the first 24-48 hours after surgery, applying ice to the operative region may help decrease swelling and relieve discomfort. Make careful to cover your skin with a towel or cloth to prevent it from coming into contact with the ice.

Elevate: When you're sleeping, elevating your legs may also aid to lessen swelling.

keep Hydrated: To keep hydrated, consume lots of fluids. However, excessive coffee and alcohol might dehydrate you and conflict with your meds.

Light Exercise: Light jogging may promote blood flow and help avoid blood clots. As directed by your surgeon, refrain from engaging in any intense activity or heavy lifting.

Healthy Eating: Eat a fibre-rich, well-balanced diet to stave against constipation. Avoid eating anything that could make you sick.

Keep a pain journal to track your pain levels and when you use painkillers. You and your healthcare practitioner may use this to evaluate your progress.

Reach out to your Surgeon: Contact your surgeon right away if you suffer any alarming symptoms, including intense or increasing pain, fever, excessive bleeding or any other symptoms.

CHAPTER 6: Dietary Considerations *(Discharged period)*

Your recovery and general health may be greatly impacted by your diet following a myomectomy. You should heed your doctor's advice and adhere to any dietary suggestions they provide.

Following a myomectomy, you should take these basic dietary precautions into account:

Hydration: Make sure you're getting enough water to stay hydrated. Constipation, a typical problem after surgery, may be avoided and recovery can be aided by proper hydration.

Foods high in Fibre: Include lots of these foods in your diet to prevent constipation and encourage regular bowel movements. Whole grains, fruits, vegetables, legumes, nuts and legume products are all good sources of fibre.

Protein: Protein plays a crucial role in tissue healing and repair. Include lean sources of protein in your meals, such as low-fat dairy, poultry, fish, tofu, beans and fowl.

Iron-rich foods: You may have been at risk for anaemia if you had previously suffered excessive monthly flow brought on by fibroids before surgery. Lean red meat, chicken, beans, lentils, spinach and fortified cereals are all iron-rich foods that you should consume to help replenish your iron levels.

Vitamin C: Helps your body absorb iron from plant-based sources and promotes the healing of wounds. Add broccoli, bell peppers, strawberries, citrus fruits and other fresh produce to your diet.

Avoid processed foods since they may cause inflammation and slow the healing process. Highly processed and sugary meals should also be avoided. Limit your consumption of processed snacks, sweetened drinks and fast meals.

Include foods with anti-inflammatory characteristics such as fatty fish *(salmon, mackerel)*, olive oil, berries, turmeric and ginger in your diet as they may help decrease inflammation and pain after surgery.

Small, Frequent meals: You may find that eating smaller, more frequent meals after surgery is more comfortable than eating larger meals. Bloating and pain may be reduced as a result.

Stay away from Alcohol and Caffeine: Both substances might slow the healing process and may interact with painkillers. During your rehabilitation, it's better to avoid or consume them in moderation.

Take notice of your body: Observe the messages coming from your body. Consider avoiding specific meals until you are completely well if they give you pain, gas, or bloating.

Medication interactions: If you're taking any
prescription drugs following a myomectomy, talk
to your doctor about any possible food
interactions or dietary considerations that could
be necessary.

Gradual return to usual food: Depending on the
complexity of the procedure and your personal
recovery, you may need to start with a bland or
soft diet before resuming your regular diet. In this
respect, heed the advice of your doctor.

CHAPTER 7: Rest, Activity Levels and Wound Care

The following basic recommendations for rest, activity levels and wound care after a myomectomy:

Recuperation and Rest:

Hospital Stay: The duration of your hospital stay will be determined by the kind of myomectomy done and how well you recover personally. It might be anywhere between a few hours and a few days.

Rest: After being released from the hospital, schedule time to recover at home for at least the first week. Avoid engaging in physically demanding activities during this time; your body needs to repair.

For the purpose of treating any discomfort, your doctor will recommend painkillers. Do not wait until the pain is unbearable to take them; rather, take them as advised.

Levels of Activity:

Walking is suggested as soon as you feel capable, which is often a day or two following surgery. It increases circulation and aids in preventing blood clots.

Strenuous Activities: For at least six weeks, or as directed by your doctor, refrain from strenuous activities including heavy lifting *(anything above 10-15 pounds)*. The healing process will be slowed down by these activities, which might pressure your incision site.

Driving: You shouldn't start until you feel confident and comfortable behind the wheel. Depending on your recuperation, this might take a few weeks.

Wound Care:

Incision care: Keep the area around the incision clean and dry. On how to take care of it, your surgeon will provide you detailed instructions. Although some redness and swelling around the incision site are normal, if you observe any infection-related symptoms *(increased redness, warmth or pus)*, you should get in touch with your doctor very once.

Staples vs stitches In a follow-up session, typically one to two weeks after your surgery, your surgeon will remove any stitches or staples you may have. Expect some scarring, but it should go away with time. Avoid placing the incision in the sun's direct rays and think about using silicone sheeting or scar treatments, as your doctor may advise, to lessen scarring.

Bathing: Normally, you can start taking showers after a few days, but you shouldn't start taking baths or going swimming until your doctor gives the all-clear.

Diet: Keep yourself hydrated by consuming plenty of liquids.

Fibre: Consuming a diet high in fibre may help reduce constipation, a side effect of both surgery and painkillers.

Be present for all planned follow-up consultations with your surgeon to track your recovery and resolve any issues; also prescription drugs should be taken as directed, including painkillers and any additional drugs your doctor may suggest for your particular situation.

Managing Discomfort

Discomfort/Pain management is crucial for a faster recovery after a myomectomy. Patients should take prescribed painkillers, engage in rest and light exercise. Maintain wound cleanliness to prevent infections and use cold packs to relieve swelling. A balanced diet and adequate water intake also aid in recovery. Consultation with medical personnel is essential for addressing any issues and maintaining a successful recovery process.

CHAPTER 8: Gradual Resumption of Activity

Recommended Exercises

After a myomectomy, it's essential to gradually get back into physical activity to guarantee a safe and successful recovery. Your post-myomectomy exercise routine should be tailored to your individual needs and should be approved by your healthcare provider. *Some general guidelines and recommended exercises for post-myomectomy recovery are:*

Start with a Walk: Begin with short, leisurely walks and gradually increase the duration and intensity. Walking helps improve circulation, reduce the risk of blood clots and aids in overall recovery.

Deep Breathing: Perform deep breathing exercises to prevent lung complications and improve oxygen flow in your body. Inhale deeply through your nose, hold for a few seconds, and exhale slowly through your mouth.

Kegels: These exercises can help strengthen your pelvic muscles and improve bladder control. To do Kegels, contract and hold your pelvic muscles for a few seconds, then release. Repeat this several times throughout the day.

Gentle Stretching: Incorporate gentle stretching exercises to improve flexibility and prevent muscle stiffness. Focus on stretches for your neck, shoulders, arms and legs.

Core Strengthening: Once your healthcare provider approves, you can start with light core-strengthening exercises. Avoid sit-ups or crunches initially, as they may put too much strain on your abdominal muscles. Instead, try exercises like pelvic tilts or modified planks.

Yoga or Pilates: These low-impact exercises can help improve flexibility and core strength. Choose classes or routines that are specifically designed for beginners or individuals recovering from surgery.

Swimming: If your incisions have healed, swimming can be an excellent low-impact exercise. It provides a full-body workout while being gentle on your joints.

Stationary Cycling: Once you're well into your recovery, stationary cycling can help improve cardiovascular fitness without putting too much stress on your abdominal muscles.

Resistance Band Exercises: Incorporate resistance band exercises for upper and lower body strength training. These can be done while sitting or lying down initially and can gradually progress to standing exercises.

Listen to Your Body: Pay close attention to how your body responds to exercise. If you experience pain, discomfort or unusual symptoms, stop the exercise immediately and consult your healthcare provider.

Start slowly and progress gradually as your body heals. It's essential to follow the guidance of your healthcare provider.

Also attend any recommended physical therapy sessions to ensure a safe and effective recovery. Prioritise safety and avoid exercises that strain your abdominal muscles until you've received clearance from your doctor.

Avoiding Strain and Heavy Lifting

These are some tips to help you stay away from strain and heavy lifting during your recovery period:

Listen to your doctor: Your surgeon will give you specific instructions for your post-operative care. It's important to follow these instructions carefully, as they will be tailored to your individual case and the type of myomectomy you had.

Restrict Physical Activity: For the first few weeks after surgery, it's important to limit your physical activity. Avoid any activities that involve heavy lifting, strenuous exercise or vigorous movement. This includes not lifting anything heavier than a few pounds.

Gradually Increase Activity: As you recover, you can slowly increase your activity level, but always follow your doctor's advice. Start with light activities like short walks and only progress to more strenuous activities when given the okay by your healthcare provider.

Wear Supportive Garments: Your surgeon may suggest wearing a support garment like an abdominal binder to give extra support to the surgical area and reduce strain.

Prevent Constipation: Straining during bowel movements can put pressure on your abdominal muscles and the surgical site. To stop constipation, eat a high-fibre diet, drink plenty of water and, if needed, use stool softeners as recommended by your doctor.

Get enough Rest: Rest is essential for the healing process. Make sure to get enough sleep and avoid activities that tire you out.

Do gentle Abdominal Exercises: Once your doctor gives you the go-ahead, you can start doing gentle abdominal exercises to help strengthen your core muscles and promote healing. However, avoid any exercises that cause discomfort or strain.

Ask for help: Don't be afraid to ask for help with tasks that involve lifting heavy objects or strenuous physical activity. Friends and family can help you with chores and errands during your recovery.

Manage pain: If you experience pain or discomfort, take prescribed pain medications as directed by your doctor. Pain can limit your mobility and increase the risk of strain, so it's important to manage it properly.

Listen to your body: Pay attention to your body's signals. If you feel any discomfort or pain when doing an activity, stop immediately and rest. Pushing through discomfort can lead to strain and slow down the healing process.

It's essential to keep in touch with your doctor and follow their instructions during the healing period after a myomectomy. The amount of time it takes to recover can differ depending on the type of myomectomy and individual factors. To reduce the risk of strain and ensure a successful recovery, it's important to take it easy, listen to your doctor's advice and prioritise your health.

CHAPTER 9: Diet and Nutrition

Post-Operative Diet

It's essential to have a healthy diet after a myomectomy to help your body heal and reduce the risk of complications.

Here are some dietary tips to follow during your recovery:

Stay hydrated by drinking plenty of water; gradually start eating again, beginning with clear liquids and light, easily digestible foods; include high-fibre foods to prevent constipation; incorporate lean sources of protein for tissue repair; consume foods rich in vitamins and minerals; add omega-3 fatty acids to your diet; avoid high-fat, fried and spicy foods; eat small, frequent meals; limit sugar and processed foods; follow your doctor's recommendations; be aware of food allergies or sensitivities; and limit alcohol and caffeine.

Details Why:

Keep hydrated

To keep hydrated, drink lots of water. Drinking enough water is essential for general recovery and to help avoid constipation, which is often experienced after surgery.

Gradually Start Eating Again:

Following your surgeon's instructions, you may begin with clear liquids and work your way up to solid meals as tolerated. Start with light, simple meals like yoghurt or gelatin, clear soups and broths.

Fibre-Rich Foods:

Consume meals rich in fibre to avoid constipation, which may put stress on your abdominal muscles. Whole grains, fruits, veggies and legumes are all healthy food options.

Healthy Proteins

Include lean sources of protein in your diet, such as skinless chicken, fish, lean meat cuts, tofu, legumes and low-fat dairy items. Protein is necessary for both general healing and tissue repair.

Nutrient-dense Foods:

To help your immune system and healing process, eat meals high in vitamins and minerals. Fruits and vegetables may be healthy, especially those that include zinc and vitamin C.

Fatty Acids Omega-3

Include foods high in omega-3 fatty acids such as flaxseeds, chia seeds, walnuts and fatty fish *(trout, salmon, mackerel)*. Omega-3 fatty acids contain anti-inflammatory qualities that help speed up recovery.

Avoid Fried, High-fat and Spicy Foods:

Fried and high-fat meals may be uncomfortable and difficult to digest. It's advised to stay away from spicy meals during the first stage of healing since they might irritate your digestive system.

Little, Regular Meals:

Consider eating smaller, more regular meals throughout the day rather than three big meals. This may provide a continuous supply of energy and assist avoid overeating.

Limit Processed Foods and Sugar:

Reduce your intake of processed meals and sugary snacks since they might cause energy spikes and crashes that might not be beneficial for healing.

Pay Attention to Your Doctor's Advice:

Depending on your unique requirements and the kind of myomectomy you had, your surgeon could have special dietary recommendations. Make sure to carefully heed their advice.

Keep an eye out for Food Sensitivity or Allergies:

Reintroducing certain foods into your diet after surgery should only be done with caution if you are aware of any food allergies or sensitivities. Additional pain and consequences might result from allergic responses.

Reduce Caffeine and Alcohol:

Caffeine and alcohol may interact with certain drugs and slow the healing process. Limiting or avoiding these drugs is advised until you are completely healed.

POST MYOMECTOMY BREAKFAST, LUNCH AND DINNER MEALS OPTION

BREAKFAST MEALS:

Oatmeal: Start with plain oatmeal and sweeten it with honey or a bit of maple syrup. Add sliced bananas, berries or chopped nuts for extra flavour and nutrition.

Greek Yoghurt Parfait: Layer Greek yoghurt with granola and fresh fruit like strawberries, blueberries, or peaches for a protein, fibre and probiotic boost.

Scrambled Eggs: Scrambled eggs are easy on the stomach and full of protein. Mix in some chopped spinach, tomatoes, and a sprinkle of cheese for a tasty twist.

Smoothie: Blend spinach, banana, frozen berries, Greek yoghurt and a scoop of protein powder or chia seeds for a nutrient-packed smoothie.

Avocado Toast: Mash ripe avocado on whole-grain toast and top with sliced tomatoes, a sprinkle of salt and pepper and a drizzle of olive oil for healthy fats and fibre.

Cottage Cheese Bowl: Combine cottage cheese with sliced peaches or pineapple. Add a drizzle of honey and some crushed nuts for extra flavour and texture.

Nut Butter and Banana Sandwich: Spread almond or peanut butter on whole-grain bread and add banana slices for a potassium-rich snack.

Quinoa Breakfast Bowl: Cook quinoa and mix it with Greek yoghurt, honey and your favourite fruit for a protein-packed breakfast.

Rice Porridge (Congee): For a warm and comforting breakfast, make rice porridge by simmering rice in broth or water until it's soft. Add shredded chicken, ginger and a touch of soy sauce for flavour.

Chia Pudding: Combine chia seeds with almond milk, a bit of honey, and some vanilla extract. Let it sit in the fridge overnight and in the morning, top it with your favourite fruits for a delicious breakfast.

Lunch Meals:

Grilled Chicken Salad: A delicious grilled chicken breast served atop a bed of mixed greens with a variety of colourful veggies like tomatoes, cucumbers, bell peppers, and carrots. Drizzle a light vinaigrette dressing over the top for a tasty finish.

Quinoa and Roasted Vegetable Bowl: Cooked quinoa combined with roasted veggies *(such as broccoli, sweet potatoes and zucchini)* and a splash of olive oil and lemon juice. Add some chickpeas or beans for an extra protein boost.

Salmon and Asparagus: Bake or grill a salmon fillet and pair it with roasted asparagus and a side of quinoa or brown rice. Squeeze some fresh lemon juice and herbs over the top for a flavorful touch.

Veggie Stir-Fry: Stir-fry a mix of colourful vegetables like bell peppers, broccoli, snap peas, and carrots in a light, low-sodium sauce. Serve it over brown rice or whole wheat noodles with tofu or lean protein of your choice.

Turkey and Avocado Wrap: Fill a whole-grain wrap with sliced turkey breast, avocado, spinach or lettuce, and a smear of hummus or Greek yoghurt as a creamy spread.

Miso Soup with Tofu and Seaweed: Enjoy a warm bowl of miso soup with added tofu and seaweed for a nutritious and comforting meal. Serve it with a side of steamed brown rice or a small salad.

Sweet Potato and Black Bean Salad: Roast some sweet potato cubes and mix them with black beans, corn, red onion and a light lime dressing. Sprinkle some chopped cilantro on top for a flavorful finish.

Lentil and Vegetable Soup: Make a homemade lentil soup with carrots, celery and spinach for a hearty and nutritious meal. Lentils are a great source of protein and fibre.

Egg Salad Sandwich: Make a healthier egg salad with Greek yoghurt instead of mayonnaise. Put it on whole-grain bread and add lettuce and tomato slices for a delicious sandwich.

Sushi Rolls: If you're a fan of sushi, opt for rolls with fresh fish, avocado and veggies. Choose brown rice or quinoa as a healthier base and use low-sodium soy sauce for dipping.

Tuna and White Bean Salad: Mix canned tuna, white beans, cherry tomatoes, red onion and parsley. Dress it with olive oil and lemon juice for a protein-packed salad.

Baked Sweet Potatoes with Cottage Cheese: Bake sweet potatoes and top them with a dollop of cottage cheese and a sprinkle of cinnamon or a drizzle of honey for a comforting and nutritious lunch.

Mushroom and Spinach Omelette: Make an omelette with sautéed mushrooms, spinach and a sprinkle of low-fat cheese. Serve it with a side of whole-grain toast or a small salad.

Hummus and Veggie Platter: Put together a colourful plate with hummus as the centrepiece, surrounded by sliced cucumbers, cherry tomatoes, baby carrots and bell pepper strips for dipping.

Tofu and Vegetable Kebabs: Skewer cubes of tofu with a variety of marinated vegetables like bell peppers, onions and zucchini. Grill or roast them for a flavorful and protein-rich meal.

Brown Rice Bowl with Beans: Mix brown rice with your choice of cooked beans *(black beans, kidney beans, or chickpeas)*, sautéed spinach or kale and a drizzle of tahini dressing.

Fruit and Nut Salad: Combine your favourite fruits, such as berries, apples and grapes, with nuts like almonds or walnuts. Add a sprinkle of feta cheese or Greek yoghurt for creaminess.

Dinner Meals:

Grilled Chicken Breast with Quinoa and Steamed Vegetables:

This meal is a great way to get lean protein from the chicken breast, complex carbohydrates and protein from quinoa and essential vitamins and minerals from steamed vegetables like broccoli, carrots, and spinach.

Baked Salmon with Brown Rice and Asparagus:

Salmon is a great choice for this meal, as it is rich in omega-3 fatty acids which can help reduce inflammation. Brown rice provides fibre and sustained energy, while asparagus is a good source of vitamins and minerals.

Vegetable Stir-Fry with Tofu and Brown Rice:

Tofu is a great plant-based protein option, and the stir-fry is packed with nutrients from a variety of colourful vegetables like bell peppers, broccoli, and snap peas. Brown rice compliments the meal with fibre and essential nutrients.

Turkey and Vegetable Soup:

Turkey is a lean protein option and a homemade vegetable soup with carrots, celery and onions is both soothing and nutritious.

Spinach and Feta Stuffed Portobello Mushrooms:

Portobello mushrooms are a great source of vitamins and minerals, and spinach and feta provide flavour and nutrients. Serve with a side salad for added greens.

Baked Sweet Potato with Black Beans and Avocado:

Sweet potatoes are packed with vitamins and fibre, black beans offer protein and fibre while avocado adds healthy fats and creaminess.

Pasta Primavera with Whole Wheat Pasta:

Whole wheat pasta is a great choice for added fibre and you can load up on colourful vegetables

like cherry tomatoes, zucchini and bell peppers.
Use a light olive oil and herb-based sauce for
flavour.

Greek Salad with Grilled Shrimp:

A Greek salad with cucumbers, tomatoes, olives
and feta cheese is a great option and you can top
it with grilled shrimp for protein. Dress with olive
oil and lemon juice for a delicious and nutritious
meal.

Lentil and Vegetable Curry with Brown Rice:

This delicious dish is a great source of plant-based
protein and iron. It's made with tomatoes, onions
and spinach, which provide vitamins and
antioxidants. Serve it with brown rice for a
complete meal.

Grilled Tofu and Vegetable Skewers with Quinoa:

Tofu and vegetables are a great combination for a
protein-packed meal. Marinate them in a light,

low-sodium sauce and serve with quinoa for a complete protein source.

Baked Cod with Roasted Brussels Sprouts and Mashed Cauliflower:

Cod is a lean fish that's full of protein and omega-3 fatty acids. Roasted Brussels sprouts and mashed cauliflower make a tasty side dish that's low in carbs.

Chickpea and Spinach Curry with Basmati Rice:

Chickpeas and spinach are a great combination for a nutritious curry. Serve it with basmati rice for a complete meal.

Oven-Roasted Turkey Breast with Steamed Green Beans and Quinoa:

Turkey breast is a lean and protein-packed option. Serve it with steamed green beans and quinoa for a balanced meal.

Miso Soup with Sushi Rolls:

Miso soup is a light and nutritious meal. Add some sushi rolls with cooked fish or vegetarian options for a complete meal.

Eggplant Parmesan with a Side Salad:

Baked eggplant is a healthy alternative to fried. Top it with tomato sauce and mozzarella cheese and serve with a side salad of mixed greens for a delicious meal.

Baked or Grilled Chicken Thighs with Sweet Potato Fries and Steamed Broccoli:

Chicken thighs are a flavorful and moist option. Serve them with sweet potato fries and steamed broccoli for a nutritious meal.

HYDRATION

Staying hydrated after a myomectomy is essential for a successful recovery. Your healthcare provider will give you specific instructions on how to stay hydrated, but *here are some general tips to keep in mind:*

Drink 8-10 cups *(64-80 ounces)* of water per day, unless your healthcare provider recommends a different amount. Clear fluids like water, clear broths or electrolyte drinks are best in the immediate hours following surgery.

Avoid caffeine and alcohol, as they can dehydrate your body. Monitor your urine colour and frequency, as clear to light yellow urine is a sign of good hydration. Sip fluids steadily throughout the day and use a straw if you have difficulty sitting up or moving. Watch for signs of dehydration, such as dry mouth, dark urine, dizziness, rapid heartbeat, or a decrease in urination.

Eating a balanced diet with fruits and vegetables can also help with hydration, as they contain water and electrolytes. Lastly, if you're taking any medications post-surgery, discuss with your healthcare provider whether they might affect your hydration levels or require adjustments in your fluid intake. Everyone's hydration needs are different, so be sure to follow your doctor's instructions.

DIETARY FIBRE AND SUPPLEMENTS

It's important to talk to your healthcare provider or a registered dietitian to create a personalised nutrition plan after your myomectomy. *Here are some general guidelines to consider:*

Fibre: Whole grains, fruits with edible skins, vegetables and legumes are all great sources of fibre. If you have trouble meeting your fibre needs through food alone, your healthcare provider may recommend a fibre supplement.

Iron: Some women may experience mild anaemia due to blood loss during surgery, so your healthcare provider may recommend iron supplements.

Calcium and Vitamin D: Make sure you're getting enough of these to support bone health, especially if you've been prescribed medications like GnRH analogs.

Protein: Include lean protein sources like poultry, fish, tofu, legumes and low-fat dairy products in your diet.

Hydration: Drink plenty of water to stay hydrated and help prevent constipation.

Limit your consumption of caffeine and alcohol, as they can interfere with your body's ability to heal and may worsen any digestive issues.

Portion Control: Be mindful of portion sizes to prevent excessive weight gain during recovery.

Gradual Changes: Make dietary changes gradually to allow your body to adjust comfortably.

Medication Considerations: Be aware that certain medications or pain relievers you are taking post-surgery might have specific dietary recommendations or restrictions. Consult your healthcare provider or pharmacist for guidance.

CHAPTER 10: Emotional and Mental Well-being

Coping with Emotions and Support Networks

EMOTIONS:

Coping with emotions after a myomectomy can be difficult. It's normal to experience a variety of emotions during the recovery process.

Here are some tips to help you manage:

Acknowledge Your Feelings: Understand that it's okay to have a mix of emotions after surgery. You may feel relief, anxiety, fear, sadness, or frustration. Allow yourself to feel these emotions without judgement.

Reach Out: Talk to your friends and family about your feelings. Sharing your emotions with those close to you can provide comfort and understanding. If you feel overwhelmed, consider talking to a therapist or counsellor who can offer professional guidance.

Educate Yourself: Learn about the myomectomy procedure and the expected recovery process. Knowing what to expect can help reduce anxiety and uncertainty.

Be Realistic: Remember that recovery takes time, and there may be ups and downs along the way. Set realistic expectations for your progress and don't rush the healing process.

Take Care of Yourself: Make sure to prioritise self-care to promote physical and emotional healing. This includes getting adequate rest, eating a balanced diet and following your doctor's recommendations for post-operative care.

Stay Active: As your doctor allows, engage in gentle physical activity like short walks. Exercise can help boost your mood and energy levels.

Mindfulness and Relaxation: Practise relaxation techniques such as deep breathing, meditation or yoga to manage stress and anxiety. These practices can help you stay calm and centred during your recovery.

Express Yourself: Consider journaling or creative outlets like art or music to express your emotions. Writing down your thoughts and feelings can be therapeutic.

Find a Support Group: Look for support groups or online communities where you can connect with others who have gone through similar experiences. Sharing your story and hearing from others can be comforting.

Focus on the Positive: Try to focus on the positive aspects of the myomectomy, such as the potential for improved health and reduced symptoms in the long run. Visualise your recovery and future well-being.

Talk to Your Healthcare Team: If you're struggling with emotional issues, don't hesitate to reach out to your healthcare team. They can provide guidance, refer you to a mental health professional if necessary or adjust your treatment plan as needed.

Emotional healing is just as important as physical healing after surgery. Be patient with yourself and give yourself the time and space to process your feelings. Over time, as you recover, your emotional well-being is likely to improve and you'll regain a sense of control and normalcy in your life.

SUPPORT NETWORKS

Having a support system is essential for those who have gone through a myomectomy. This network can provide emotional, physical and informational assistance during the healing process.

Here are some post-myomectomy support networks and resources to consider:

Family and Friends: Lean on your loved ones for emotional support, help with daily tasks and companionship during your recovery.

Online Forums and Support Groups: Join online communities, such as forums, Facebook groups or Reddit communities, that are dedicated to discussing experiences related to myomectomy. These platforms can be beneficial for sharing stories, asking questions and finding comfort in the shared experiences of others.

Local Support Groups: See if there are any local support groups or organisations that focus on women's health or gynaecological issues. They may offer in-person meetings, seminars or counselling services.

Therapist or Counselor: If you're having emotional difficulties related to your myomectomy, consider talking to a therapist or counsellor who specialises in women's health or post-surgery support.

Patient Advocacy Organisations: Organisations like the Fibroid Foundation, Endometriosis Foundation of America or the American Cancer Society can provide resources, support and information related to myomectomy and gynaecological health.

Online Health Communities: Websites like Inspire, PatientsLikeMe or HealthUnlocked offer communities for individuals dealing with various health issues, including those related to gynaecological surgeries.

Medical Professionals: Your surgical team, including your gynaecologist or surgeon, can provide guidance and support during your recovery. Don't be afraid to reach out if you have questions or concerns.

Nutritional Support: Consult with a registered dietitian or nutritionist who can help you create a healthy eating plan to support your recovery and overall well-being.

Physical Therapist: Depending on your particular case and surgery, you may benefit from physical therapy to aid in your recovery and help manage any pain or discomfort.

Books and Educational Resources: There are numerous books and online resources dedicated to women's health and myomectomy recovery. These can provide valuable information and tips.

Each individual's experience with myomectomy is different, so it's crucial to tailor your support network to your specific needs and circumstances. Reach out to multiple sources for comprehensive support and don't be afraid to ask for help when you need it.

CHAPTER 11: Follow-up Care

Post-Operative Appointments And Monitoring Healing Progress

After a myomectomy, it is essential to follow the post-operative care plan and attend follow-up appointments to ensure a successful recovery. The type of myomectomy *(abdominal, laparoscopic or hysteroscopic)* and your individual medical condition will determine the specifics of your post-operative care plan.

Below are some general guidelines for post-operative appointments following a myomectomy:

Immediately after the surgery, you will be monitored in the recovery room until you are awake and stable. Once you are transferred to your hospital room, the medical staff will continue to monitor your vital signs and manage your pain.

The length of your hospital stay will depend on the type of myomectomy and your individual recovery. Abdominal myomectomies typically require a longer hospital stay *(1-3 days)*, while laparoscopic and hysteroscopic myomectomies often allow for shorter stays *(typically overnight or less)*. Before leaving the hospital, you will receive detailed instructions on caring for your incisions, managing pain and any medications you need to take.

Your first follow-up appointment with your surgeon will typically occur about 1-2 weeks after the surgery. During this appointment, your surgeon will check your incisions, discuss your recovery progress and may remove any sutures or staples if necessary. They will also likely review the pathology report of the removed fibroids if applicable.

Depending on your surgeon's recommendations and your individual recovery, you may have additional follow-up appointments at regular intervals *(e.g., 6 weeks, 3 months, 6 months and 1 year)* to monitor your progress and address any concerns or complications.

Your surgeon will discuss expected recovery milestones with you, such as when it's safe to resume normal activities, including exercise, sexual activity and fertility-related discussions if applicable. If fertility is a concern, your surgeon may discuss your options for conceiving post-myomectomy. It's important to have these discussions with your healthcare provider if you plan to have children in the future. You may also need to discuss contraception options if you are sexually active and do not wish to become pregnant during your recovery period.

If you experience any unusual symptoms or complications during your recovery, such as heavy bleeding, signs of infection, severe pain or fever, contact your doctor immediately or seek emergency medical care. Depending on your medical history and the specifics of your myomectomy, your surgeon may recommend periodic check-ups in the years following the surgery to monitor for fibroid recurrence or other gynaecological issues.

It is important to follow your surgeon's advice and post-operative care plan to ensure a smooth recovery and the best possible outcome after a myomectomy.

Monitoring Healing Progress

It is essential to keep track of the healing process after a myomectomy to ensure a successful recovery and to detect any potential issues. Key steps and considerations to keep in mind when monitoring the healing progress:

Immediately after the surgery, you will be monitored in the recovery room to make sure you are stable. Your vital signs, such as blood pressure, heart rate and breathing, will be monitored and pain management will be initiated to keep you comfortable.

The length of your hospital stay will depend on the type of myomectomy and your individual recovery. Before you are discharged, your healthcare team will provide instructions on wound care, pain management and activity restrictions.

If you had an abdominal or laparoscopic myomectomy, you will have incisions that need to be taken care of. Make sure to keep the incisions clean and dry and follow your surgeon's instructions for changing dressings and keeping the area sterile. If you notice any signs of infection, such as increased redness, swelling, warmth or discharge from the incisions, report them to your healthcare provider.

Take prescribed pain medications as directed and gradually transition from stronger pain medications to over-the-counter pain relievers as your pain decreases.

Follow your healthcare provider's recommendations for pain management. Avoid strenuous activities, heavy lifting and vigorous exercise for the specified duration recommended by your surgeon, which is typically several weeks. Gradually increase your activity level as you feel comfortable and get plenty of rest to aid in the healing process.

Maintain a balanced diet rich in fibre, fruits, vegetables and lean protein to support healing, and stay hydrated to promote tissue repair. Attend all scheduled follow-up appointments with your surgeon or gynaecologist. During these visits, your healthcare provider will assess your healing progress, discuss any concerns and may perform pelvic exams or imaging studies if necessary. Be aware of any signs of complications, such as excessive bleeding, fever, severe abdominal pain, or unusual discharge and contact your doctor immediately if you experience any concerning symptoms.

It is common for menstrual cycle patterns to change after a myomectomy. Your periods may be lighter or heavier and you may experience changes in menstrual pain.

If you plan to conceive after a myomectomy, discuss your fertility options and timing with your healthcare provider.

Healing times can vary depending on the type of myomectomy, the number and size of fibroids removed and also individual factors.

Complications and Warning Signs

It is extremely important to be aware of potential complications and warning signs that may occur after a myomectomy. Some things to watch out for during your recovery:

Infection: Look out for fever, increased pain, redness, swelling or discharge from the incision site.

Bleeding: Some postoperative bleeding is normal, but if you soak through more than one pad an hour or notice large blood clots, seek medical attention.

Pain and Discomfort: Severe or worsening pain may be a sign of complications, such as infection, hematoma *(collection of blood at the surgical site)* or injury to nearby structures.

Fever: If your temperature rises above 100.4°F *(38°C)*, contact your healthcare provider.

Difficulty Urinating: If you are unable to urinate or experience severe pain while urinating, seek medical attention.

Constipation: Pain medications and anaesthesia can cause constipation. Stool softeners or laxatives may be recommended to prevent straining, which can be harmful to the surgical site.

Vaginal Discharge: You may have some vaginal discharge after a myomectomy, which can be bloody and is usually normal. However, if the discharge becomes foul-smelling or excessive, contact your healthcare provider.

Recovery Time: Most patients can return to normal activities within a few weeks to a few months, depending on the type of myomectomy. If you're experiencing significant delays in your recovery, consult your surgeon.

Allergic Reactions: If you experience hives, itching, swelling or difficulty breathing after taking medications prescribed for post-surgery pain or infection, seek immediate medical attention, as it may indicate an allergic reaction.

Signs of Blood Clots: Although rare, blood clots can form after surgery. Symptoms of blood clots may include sudden leg pain, swelling, warmth, redness or difficulty breathing. If you suspect a blood clot, seek immediate medical care.

Wound Dehiscence: If you notice your incision opening, contact your surgeon right away.

Adverse Reactions to Anesthesia: If you develop severe nausea, vomiting, difficulty breathing or chest pain, seek medical help immediately.

Please follow your surgeon's post-operative instructions, attend follow-up appointments and communicate any unusual or concerning symptoms promptly.

CHAPTER 12: Returning to Work and Daily Life

Timing and Planning

Before scheduling your myomectomy, it's important to discuss your recovery plan with your surgeon. Depending on the type of surgery, your overall health and the nature of your job and daily activities, the amount of time it takes to return to work and daily life after a myomectomy can vary.

- Abdominal myomectomies typically require a longer recovery time of 6 to 8 weeks.

- Laparoscopic or robotic-assisted procedures may take 2 to 6 weeks.

The length of your hospital stay will depend on the type of surgery and your individual recovery. If you have a desk job, you may be able to return to work sooner, potentially within 2 to 6 weeks, depending on your recovery progress and how you feel.

If your job involves heavy lifting or strenuous physical activity, you may need to take a more extended leave. It's essential to follow your doctor's recommendations and pay attention to your body's signals during the recovery process.

- Avoid strenuous activities, heavy lifting and vigorous exercise for the first few weeks after surgery.

- Gradually increase your activity level as your surgeon advises and listen to your body.

- Take prescribed medications as directed, attend all follow-up appointments with your surgeon and follow dietary guidelines and any restrictions on certain activities *(e.g., sexual activity)* during your recovery period.

It's also important to have a support system in place during your recovery. Family and friends can assist with daily tasks and provide emotional support. Surgery and recovery can be emotionally challenging, so don't hesitate to seek emotional support from a therapist or support group if needed. Before your surgery, plan for time off from work and daily responsibilities. Ensure you have someone to assist with household chores and childcare if necessary.

Workplace Considerations

There are a few things to consider when returning to work. Firstly, the length of your recovery will depend on the type of myomectomy you had and your overall health. It could take anywhere from a few weeks to several months. During the initial postoperative period, you will likely need to take some time off work to allow your body to heal. It is important to follow your doctor's advice regarding when it is safe for you to return to work. Make sure to communicate openly with your healthcare provider about your job requirements and any worries you have related to your return to work.

It is also important to understand your physical limitations during the recovery period. Activities that involve heavy lifting or strenuous physical exertion may be restricted for some time.

Talk to your doctor about your job responsibilities to determine if any modifications are necessary to accommodate your recovery. Pain and discomfort are common after a myomectomy, so your doctor may prescribe pain medication. Be aware of the side effects of pain medication and discuss these with your doctor.

Fatigue is normal during the recovery process, so you may need to take breaks, rest or adjust your work hours to manage fatigue. Let your employer know about your need for flexibility during this time.

Additionally, evaluate your work environment for potential stressors and factors that may impact your recovery. Discuss any necessary changes with your employer, such as ergonomic adjustments or workload modifications.

It is also important to build a support system at work. Let your colleagues or supervisor know about your surgery and recovery timeline so they can provide assistance or adjust work expectations if needed. Depending on your surgery and your mode of transportation to work, you may need to arrange for assistance with commuting during your recovery.

Lastly, keep your follow-up appointments with your healthcare provider to monitor your progress. Be prepared to discuss any work-related concerns during these appointments.

Resuming Normal Activities

After a myomectomy, it's important to plan and consider your individual recovery process before resuming normal activities. The timeline for returning to regular activities can depend on the type of myomectomy you had *(laparoscopic, abdominal, hysteroscopic)*, the size and number of fibroids removed and your overall health.

It's essential to follow your doctor's post-operative instructions, as they will provide personalised guidance based on your specific situation.

Some general guidelines to help you plan your recovery:

Immediately after the Procedure (O-2 weeks):

- Rest and recuperation are key during the first few days after surgery. You may need to stay in the hospital for a day or two, depending on the type and complexity of the myomectomy.

- Pain management is important during this period, and your doctor will prescribe appropriate pain medications. Avoid strenuous physical activities, heavy lifting and driving during this phase.

- Gradually introduce light walking to promote circulation and prevent blood clots.

2-4 weeks after Surgery:

As you start to recover, you can gradually increase your activity level, but avoid high-impact exercises, lifting heavy objects and vigorous physical activities.

Continue taking any prescribed pain medications as needed. Pay attention to your body and if you experience excessive bleeding, fever or severe pain, contact your healthcare provider immediately.

You may still need assistance with certain daily tasks, so have a support system in place.

4-6 weeks after Surgery:

By this time, you should be able to resume light to moderate activities, such as light exercise *(e.g., walking, gentle yoga)* and gradually increasing your mobility. Consult with your doctor before resuming sexual activity or using tampons.

Continue to attend your post-operative follow-up appointments for monitoring and any necessary adjustments to your recovery plan.

6+ weeks after Surgery:

Around 6-8 weeks after the surgery, you should be able to resume most normal activities, including driving, lifting heavier objects and returning to work. However, consult with your doctor for personalised advice. It's essential to continue monitoring your symptoms and if you experience any unusual discomfort or complications, contact your healthcare provider promptly.

CHAPTER 13: Fertility and Pregnancy After Myomectomy

Discussing Fertility Goals

After a myomectomy, discussing reproductive objectives is a crucial and sometimes difficult dialogue that includes the patient and their medical professional. Uterine fibroids are benign growths that may sometimes affect fertility. When talking about reproductive objectives after a myomectomy, keep the following considerations in mind:

Meeting with a Specialist:

After a myomectomy, it's critical to speak with a medical professional who focuses on fertility or reproductive medicine. They may evaluate your particular condition, taking into account the size and location of the fibroids, the kind of myomectomy done, as well as your general health.

Myomectomy timing

The myomectomy's timing may have an effect on fertility. Your chances of becoming pregnant may increase if the fibroids were interfering with your fertility. But myomectomy type and the degree of tissue damage caused by the procedure may also have an impact on fertility.

Recuperation and Healing:

It's important to give your body time to recuperate and mend after a myomectomy before trying to become pregnant. When it's safe to begin attempting to become pregnant will be determined by your healthcare practitioner.

Fertility Evaluation:

A semen analysis for your spouse *(if appropriate)* as well as blood tests to examine hormone levels and ultrasounds to monitor ovarian and uterine health are just a few of the reproductive tests that your doctor could advise. Your reproductive status may be determined with the use of these tests.

Options for Treatment:

Your doctor may recommend a number of treatments, depending on the severity of your fibroids and any reproductive problems. They could consist of:

- **Natural pregnancy** is possible if the fibroids were effectively removed by the myomectomy and no other reproductive problems exist.

- **Assisted reproductive technologies *(ART)*:** In certain circumstances, ART techniques like in vitro fertilisation *(IVF)* may be advised to increase your chances of becoming pregnant.

- **Medication:** To increase fertility, control your menstrual cycle or reduce any residual fibroids, your doctor may recommend medication.

- **A repeat myomectomy** can be required if the fibroids recur or if not all of them were removed during the previous procedure.

Threats and Complications:

Discuss possible hazards and issues related to reproductive treatments, such as the potential for ART to result in multiple pregnancies or fibroid recurrence.

Support for the soul:

It may be emotionally difficult to deal with reproductive issues. Seek out friends, relatives, support groups or a therapist who can provide you understanding and encouragement.

Living Conditions

Fertility may be impacted by lifestyle choices including managing stress, keeping a healthy weight, quitting smoking and drinking too much alcohol. Your doctor could provide advice on modifying your way of living.

Transparent Communication:

Throughout your path towards becoming pregnant, be honest and open with your healthcare provider. Ask questions, voice your concerns and work with others to choose the best course of action.

Addressing your reproductive objectives following a myomectomy is a personalised procedure that should take into consideration your particular medical background and situation. Seek advice from a reproductive medicine expert and be ready for a thorough examination to establish the best strategy for attaining your fertility objectives.

Pregnancy Planning and Monitoring

Planning and monitoring a pregnancy after a myomectomy is an essential process to ensure a healthy pregnancy and reduce potential complications.

Here are some key steps and considerations for those who have had a myomectomy and are either planning to become pregnant or are already pregnant:

Before Pregnancy:

- Before trying to conceive, make an appointment with your obstetrician/gynaecologist (OB/GYN) or fertility specialist. Talk about your medical history, the specifics of your myomectomy and any worries you may have about fertility or pregnancy.

- It's essential to give your body enough time to heal after the myomectomy. The recommended waiting period varies depending on the type of myomectomy and the extent of the surgery, but it's usually around 3 to 6 months.

- If you are concerned about your fertility, your healthcare provider may suggest fertility testing to assess your reproductive health. This may include assessing your ovarian reserve, checking fallopian tube patency and evaluating your partner's fertility as well.

- If you have any underlying medical conditions or factors that could affect your pregnancy, such as polycystic ovary syndrome (PCOS) or diabetes, work with your healthcare provider to manage these conditions properly before conception.

- Start taking prenatal vitamins that contain folic acid at least three months before conception. Folic acid is essential for foetal development and can help prevent neural tube defects.

During Pregnancy:

Regular Prenatal Care: As soon as you confirm your pregnancy, make an appointment with your healthcare provider to begin prenatal care. Regular check-ups and monitoring are essential to ensure the health of both you and your baby.

Discuss Surgical Details: Give your healthcare provider the details of your myomectomy, such as the type of surgery, location of the fibroids and any complications that occurred during or after the procedure. This information can help guide your prenatal care and monitor potential issues.

Ultrasound and Imaging: Your healthcare provider may suggest periodic ultrasounds or other imaging studies to monitor the growth and position of any remaining fibroids and to check on the developing foetus.

High-Risk Pregnancy Evaluation: Depending on the specifics of your myomectomy and any complications that occurred during or after surgery, your pregnancy may be considered high-risk. In such cases, your healthcare provider may suggest additional monitoring and consultations with a maternal-foetal medicine specialist.

Pain and Discomfort: Some women may experience abdominal discomfort or pain during pregnancy due to the presence of scar tissue from the myomectomy. Talk to your healthcare provider about any pain or discomfort for appropriate management.

After Pregnancy:

Discuss your delivery options with your healthcare provider. In some cases, a caesarean section *(C-section)* may be recommended if there is concern about fibroids obstructing the birth canal or causing other complications.

After giving birth, your healthcare provider may continue to monitor any remaining fibroids to make sure they don't cause issues in the postpartum period.

Family Planning: If you plan to have more children, talk to your healthcare provider about your family planning goals. They can provide guidance on the timing of subsequent pregnancies and any necessary precautions.

Conclusion

LOOKING TOWARD THE FUTURE

It's critical to act proactively to guarantee a bright and healthy future after a myomectomy.

Following your doctor's instructions, allowing for recovery time, managing pain and discomfort.

Easing back into regular activities gradually, eating a healthy diet, keeping an eye on your symptoms, talking to your doctor about fertility and family planning.

Getting regular follow-up care, managing your emotional well-being, talking about contraception options, changing your lifestyle and staying informed are all part of this. A lot of individuals go on to enjoy healthy, productive lives with the correct support and care.

I Wish You Healthy, Safe And Full Recovery!

Check out our Related publication

Low Sugar Diet For Fibroids And Hormonal Imbalance

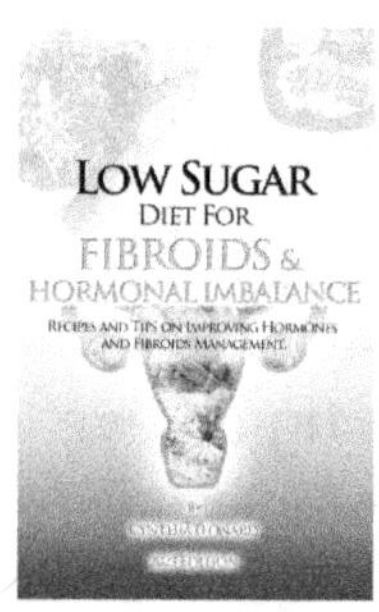